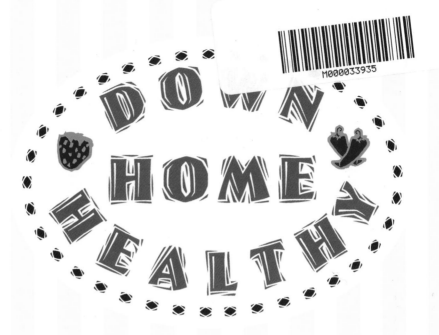

DOWN HOME HEALTHY

Family Recipes of Black American Chefs

Leah Chase

and

Johnny Rivers

National Cancer Institute
National Heart, Lung, and Blood Institute
U.S. DEPARTMENT OF HEALTH
AND HUMAN SERVICES
Public Health Service
National Institutes of Health

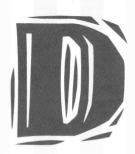

DEAR READERS:

Things sure aren't what they were. When we were kids, growing up with our brothers and sisters, we thought nothing of getting up before dawn to walk miles along back country roads picking wild blackberries or going to the little fresh vegetable market and buying butter beans and mustards and then back the many miles to a big breakfast. We didn't eat standing up or in a rush; we all sat at the table, savoring the food and the warmth of the kitchen. Then it was off again to help with the chores or on the long walk to school and back. Those were considered healthy habits.

Nowadays, who walks any distance or eats with the care we did? Now, it seems that our modern lifestyle contributes to ill health; that we exercise too little and eat too much of the wrong things and that this contributes to our getting sick. What's more, statistics tell us that black folks have a higher than average risk compared to others of getting heart disease, cancer and other diet-related diseases and dying from them. Now that's bad news. But those same health professionals tell us there's something we can do to help change that, and that's the good news. We can eat right. And that doesn't mean giving up our wonderful "soul food." Not at all. By making the right food choices for ourselves and our kids when we cook "down home-style," we can reduce the risk of getting those diseases in the first place. That's pretty important information. We're concerned and, in our small way, we feel we can help. The health folks have told us *what* to do, we'd like to help show you *how* to do it.

F I R S T, follow *the Dietary Guidelines for Americans**

- Eat a variety of foods.
- Maintain healthy weight.
- Choose a diet low in fat, saturated fat, and cholesterol.
- Choose a diet with plenty of vegetables, fruits, and grain products.
- Use sugars only in moderation.
- Use salt and sodium only in moderation.
- If you drink alcoholic beverages, do so in moderation.

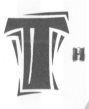**T H E N,** follow our recipes and hints, which will help you follow the dietary guidelines. We like to think they'll help start you on the road to good health.

Here's to your health and happiness.

Leah Chase
Chef & Proprietor
Dooky Chase's Restaurant
New Orleans, Louisiana

Johnny Rivers, C.E.C., A.A.C.
Executive Chef, Resorts
Walt Disney World
Orlando, Florida

* for a copy of the *Dietary Guidelines for Americans*, contact the Consumer Information Center, Department 514-4, Pueblo, Colorado 81009.

LEAH CHASE

Born in New Orleans in 1923, Leah was reared in a little town across the lake called Madisonville, Louisiana. She was the top of the line of eleven children and though while growing up, she'd do "anything to keep out of the kitchen," she learned all she knows by watching her mother and sisters whip up the family meals. Most of what the Chase family ate came from the rich variety of vegetables Leah's daddy grew in the family garden. In 1942, at the age of eighteen, Leah returned to New Orleans and found herself waiting tables in the French Quarter of the city. Not only did Leah love it, she wanted to own and run her own restaurant. "I didn't intend to do any cooking at first," Leah remembers, "but, you see, I had so many ideas in my head about food and what to serve, and I've been in the kitchen ever since." Her creative cuisine and legendary Creole gumbo made Dooky Chase's, her family-owned restaurant, into a national treasure. She uses her skill and experience to toss together the cultures of the French, the Spanish, a little American Indian and African into her pot. "You have to put all your love in that pot," says the master chef. Leah attributes the good health of her family to the limited meat in their diet. "We were poor, but my mother never had any sick children because when we were coming up, the beans, the cabbage, and the greens were the mainstay. We had lots of 'em." An active member in the community, Leah often cooks up food for housing units and homeless shelters. Her only advice is not to limit your creativity by following any hard rules. "Rules don't no more make a cook than sermons make a saint," she says.

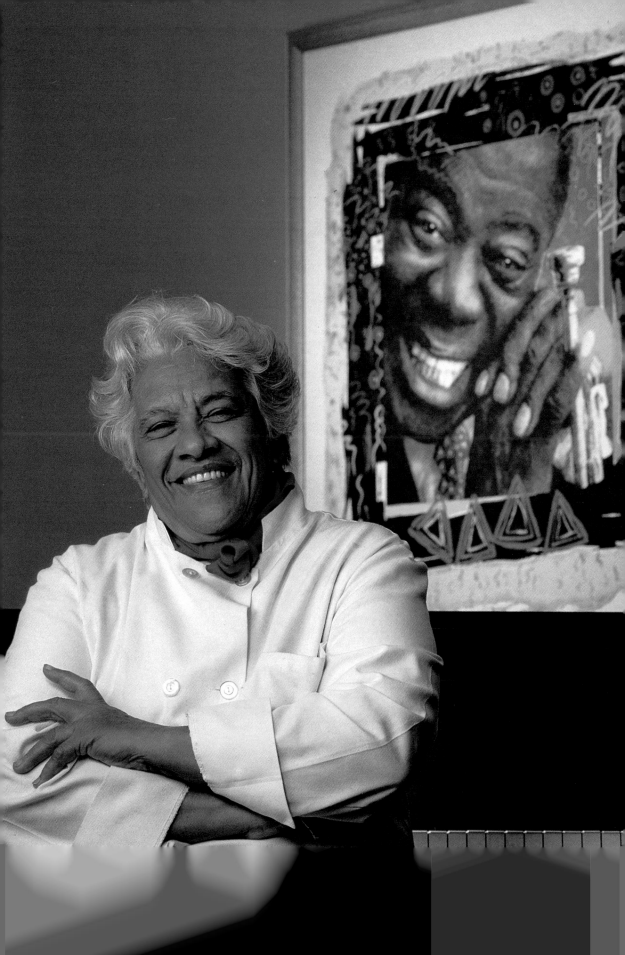

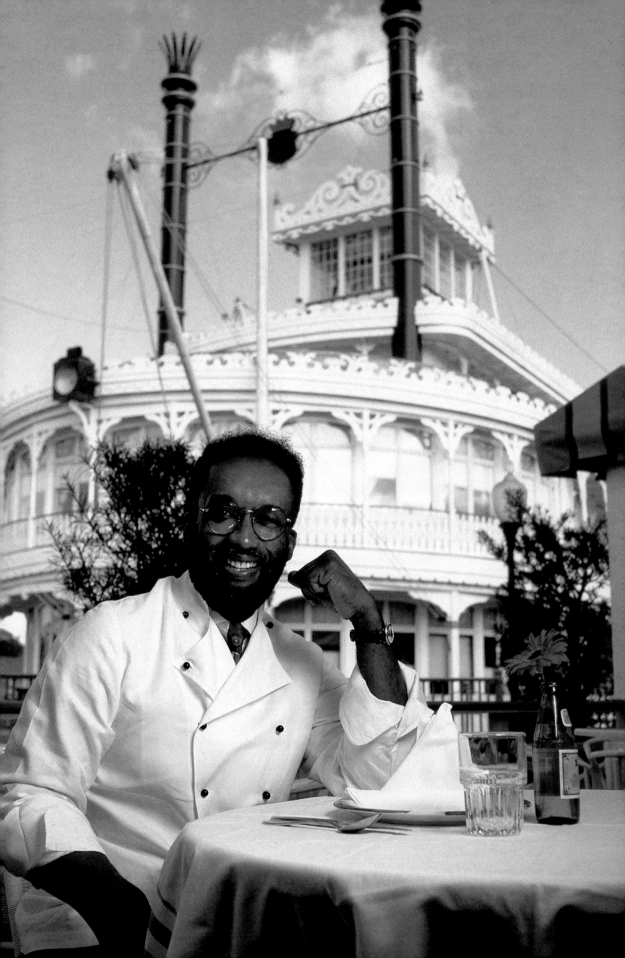

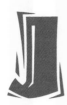# OHNNY RIVERS

If you ask him what his favorite dish is, Johnny Rivers will tell you it's "whatever I'm preparing at the time," but he wasn't always so enthusiastic about the art of cooking. Born in 1948, Johnny grew up in Orlando, Florida, where his parents were steering him toward a career in medicine. After briefly studying pre-med at Emory College, Johnny's interests turned toward the culinary arts. Ever since he was thirteen, he had worked in kitchens part-time. "I found I was pretty good at doing a lot of things with food," Johnny remembers. He also found himself captivated by the "tall chef hats and the clanging of the steel knives. And the rest is history." He traveled abroad to Europe and later across the States learning the tricks of the trade as he went. He finally settled back in Florida in 1970 and went to work for Walt Disney World Resorts. His talents and achievements as an Executive Chef with Walt Disney have since won him world fame and countless culinary awards and medals. Today, Johnny devotes much of his time lecturing and conducting seminars around the country as well as helping young people to get started in the art of cooking. He's especially concerned about the poor diet of the Black community. "We grew up through a culture eating a lot of pork and a lot of cheaper cuts of meat," Johnny says. "But now we're coming up on the year 2000 and we don't have any more excuses not to eat right. Black folks need to get serious about their diets and we can do that and have fun with it, too."

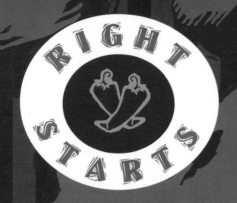

RIGHT STARTS

To play baseball, you've got to have a ball and bat. To cook lowfat, you have to have lowfat ingredients. These ingredients will help you cut back on saturated fat and cholesterol as well.

"Above all, use seasonings. Use a variety of herbs and spices instead of salt and use them often. Instead of salt in your greens, add fresh green pepper and basil. When cooking black eyed peas, add Spanish onion and crushed black pepper. Add pepper first, then taste. You'll discover a new, intense flavor in all your main dishes."
—*Leah Chase*

"Always use lowfat (1% or 2% fat), skim, nonfat dry, or evaporated skim milk for cooking instead of whole milk or cream. It makes little difference to the taste, but a big difference to your health." —*Johnny Rivers*

The key to cooking "Down Home Healthy" is to use:

Lean meats such as round, sirloin, chuck arm pot roast, loin, lean and extra lean ground beef (see list p.31) Poultry with skin removed Fish Bean and grain dishes	*instead of*	High fat meat
Skinless chicken thighs	*instead of*	Neck bone
Turkey thighs	*instead of*	Ham hocks and fatback
Small amount of vegetable oil	*instead of*	Lard, butter, or other fats that are hard at room temperature
Turkey bacon, lean ham, Canadian bacon (omit if on a low sodium diet)	*instead of*	Pork bacon
Ground skinless turkey breast	*instead of*	Pork sausage
Ground boneless turkey breast	*instead of*	Ground beef and pork
Lowfat (1% - 2%) or nonfat/skim milk	*instead of*	Whole milk
Lowfat or part skim milk cheeses	*instead of*	Whole milk cheeses
Evaporated skim milk	*instead of*	Cream
Mustard	*instead of*	Regular mayonnaise in sandwiches
Nonfat or lowfat dressing, yogurt or mayonnaise	*instead of*	Regular mayonnaise in salads and sandwiches
Fruits & vegetables without added fat	*instead of*	Avocado, olives, etc., as salad garnishes
Low sodium bouillon and broths	*instead of*	Regular bouillons and broths

Now that the cupboard is stocked, let's look at the kitchen. Put away that deep fat fryer and replace it with a steamer. Get in the mood by thinking about:

Broiling, steaming, roasting/baking, microwaving, grilling, braising/stewing, boiling, simmering, stirfrying with a little bit of oil (no more than 1-2 tablespoons oil for 4 servings)	*instead of*	Frying Basting with fat Cooking in fatty sauces and gravies

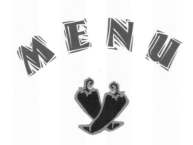

MENU

20-Minute Chicken Creole*

Garlic Mashed Potatoes*

Green Salad with Lemon Wedges

Old Fashioned Bread Pudding

Apple-Raisin Sauce

*Recipe included

"For a while, my father didn't want to raise chickens. They always seemed to get into his precious garden. Later, he relaxed a little and we enjoyed the fruits of his labors with fried chicken and chicken creole. When I discovered that frying in fat was unhealthy, I cut back. For this 'Creole,' I use no fat at all and use lots of vegetables. Tastes great!"
—*Leah Chase*

"I make my bread pudding without butter and with evaporated skim milk and egg whites now. Same rich taste, fewer calories and next to no fat. For a delicious sauce, mix cornstarch with a little water and stir it into the hot milk, sugar and seasonings mixture. You don't have to use the traditional butter and flour."
—*Leah Chase*

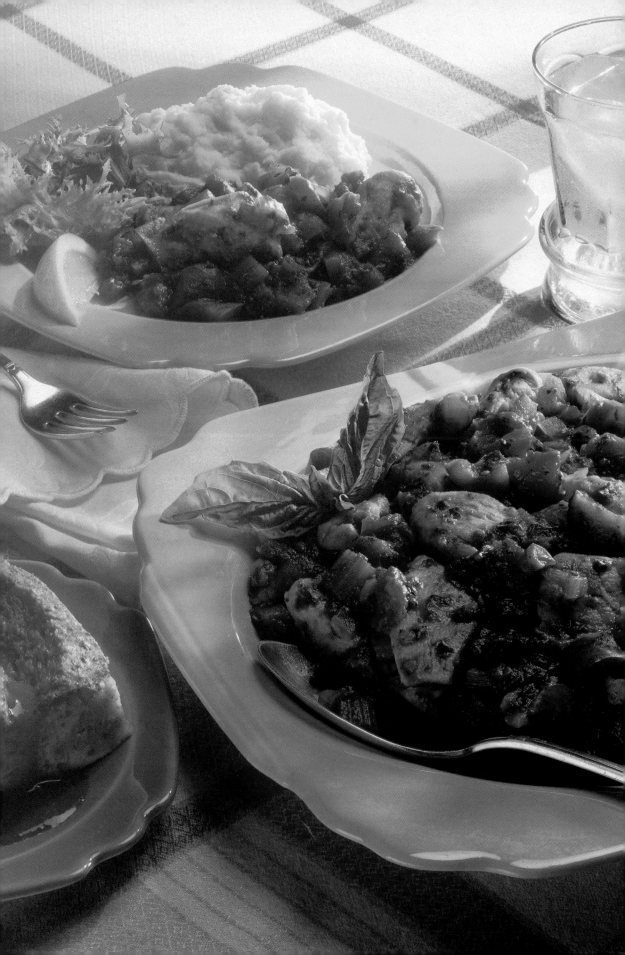

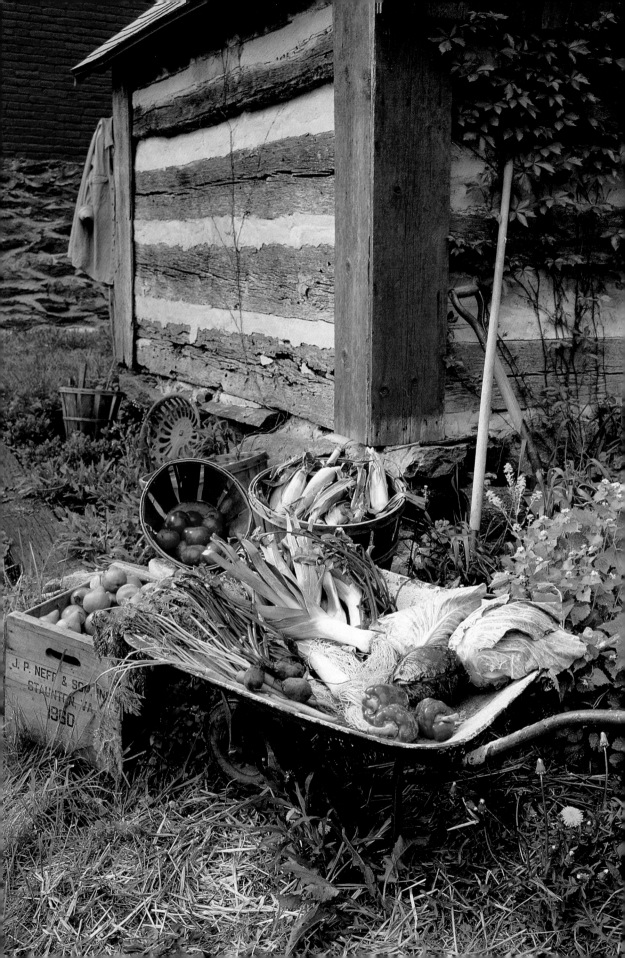

20-MINUTE CHICKEN CREOLE

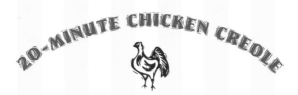

4 medium chicken breast halves (1½ lbs total), skinned, boned, and cut into 1-inch strips*

1, 14 -oz can tomatoes, cut up**

1 cup low sodium chili sauce

1½ cups chopped green pepper (1 large)

½ cup chopped celery

¼ cup chopped onion

2 cloves garlic, minced

1 tbsp chopped fresh basil or 1 tsp dried basil, crushed

1 tbsp chopped fresh parsley or 1 tsp dried parsley

¼ tsp crushed red pepper

¼ tsp salt

Nonstick spray coating

Spray deep skillet with nonstick spray coating. Preheat pan over high heat. Cook chicken in hot skillet, stirring, for 3 to 5 minutes, or until no longer pink.

Reduce heat. Add tomatoes and their juice, low sodium chili sauce, green pepper, celery, onion, garlic, basil, parsley, crushed red pepper, and salt. Bring to boiling; reduce heat and simmer, covered, for 10 minutes. Serve over hot cooked rice or whole wheat pasta.

*You can substitute 1 lb boneless, skinless, chicken breasts, cut into 1-inch strips, if desired.

**To cut back on sodium, try low sodium canned tomatoes

Makes 4 servings
Per serving:

calories: 255 total	sodium: 465 mg
fat: 3 g*	dietary fiber: 1.5 g
saturated fat: 0.8 g**	carbohydrates: 16 g
cholesterol: 100 mg**	protein: 31 g

Note: Abbreviations used throughout book include:
* g = grams
** mg = milligrams

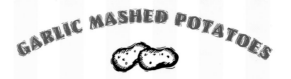

GARLIC MASHED POTATOES

1 lb potatoes (2 large)

2 cups skim milk

2 large cloves garlic, chopped

½ tsp white pepper

Peel potatoes; cut in quarters. Cook, covered, in a small amount of boiling
water for 20 to 25 minutes or until tender. Remove from heat.
Drain. Recover the pot with potatoes.

Meanwhile, in a small saucepan over low heat, cook garlic in milk until garlic is soft,
about 30 minutes.

Add milk-garlic mixture and white pepper to potatoes. Beat with an electric mixer
on low speed or mash with a potato masher until smooth.

Microwave Directions

Scrub potatoes, pat dry, and prick with a fork. On a plate, cook potatoes, uncovered,
on 100% power (high) until tender, about 12 minutes, turning potatoes over once.
Let stand 5 minutes. Peel and quarter.

Meanwhile, in a 4-cup glass measure combine milk and garlic. Cook, uncovered, on
50% power (medium) until garlic is soft, about 4 minutes.
Continue as directed above.

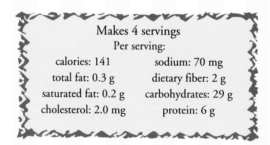

Makes 4 servings
Per serving:

calories: 141	sodium: 70 mg
total fat: 0.3 g	dietary fiber: 2 g
saturated fat: 0.2 g	carbohydrates: 29 g
cholesterol: 2.0 mg	protein: 6 g

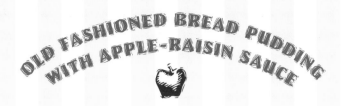

OLD FASHIONED BREAD PUDDING WITH APPLE-RAISIN SAUCE

BREAD PUDDING

10 slices whole wheat bread	1 tsp vanilla extract
1 egg	½ tsp cinnamon
3 egg whites	¼ tsp nutmeg
1½ cups skim milk	¼ tsp cloves
¼ cup sugar	2 tsp sugar
¼ cup brown sugar	

Preheat the oven to 350 F. Spray an 8x8-inch baking dish with vegetable oil spray.

Lay the slices of bread in the baking dish in two rows, overlapping them like shingles. In a medium mixing bowl, beat together the egg, egg whites, milk, ¼ cup sugar, the brown sugar and vanilla. Pour the egg mixture over the bread.

In a small bowl stir together the cinnamon, nutmeg, cloves and 2 tsp sugar. Sprinkle the spiced sugar over the bread pudding. Bake the pudding for 30 to 35 minutes, until it has browned on top and is firm to the touch.
Serve warm or at room temperature, with warm apple-raisin sauce.

APPLE-RAISIN SAUCE

1¼ cups apple juice	¼ tsp ground cinnamon
½ cup apple butter	¼ tsp ground nutmeg
2 tbsp molasses	½ tsp orange zest (optional)
½ cup raisins	

Stir all the ingredients together in a medium saucepan.
Bring to a simmer over low heat. Let the sauce simmer 5 minutes. Serve warm.
Makes 2 cups

Makes 9 servings
Per serving:

calories: 233	sodium: 252 mg
total fat: 3 g	dietary fiber: 3 g
saturated fat: 1 g	carbohydrates: 46 g
cholesterol: 24 mg	protein: 7 g

MENU

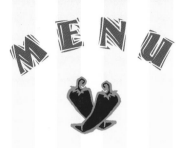

Catfish Stew and Rice*

Spinach Salad with Turkey Bacon Bits/Lowfat salad dressing

Summer Crisp*.

*Recipe included

"This is my sister Carolyn's favorite dish. She needed something that could be cooked quickly in one pot after she got home from work. The main ingredient was catfish. Since her favorite vegetable was cabbage, it seemed natural to add that to the stew, too. At my home, I some-times make this with greens instead of cabbage."

"Nutritionists say we should eat fish more often. It's relatively low in calories, low in saturated fat and total fat, a source of high-quality protein and vitamins and minerals. Any firm fleshed fish would be delicious; a low-priced fish, like grouper, catfish, or monkfish, would be easier on the pocketbook. Another simple way of using more fish in your menus is to oven bake it, following the recipe for the Baked Pork Chops on page 27.
— *Johnny Rivers*

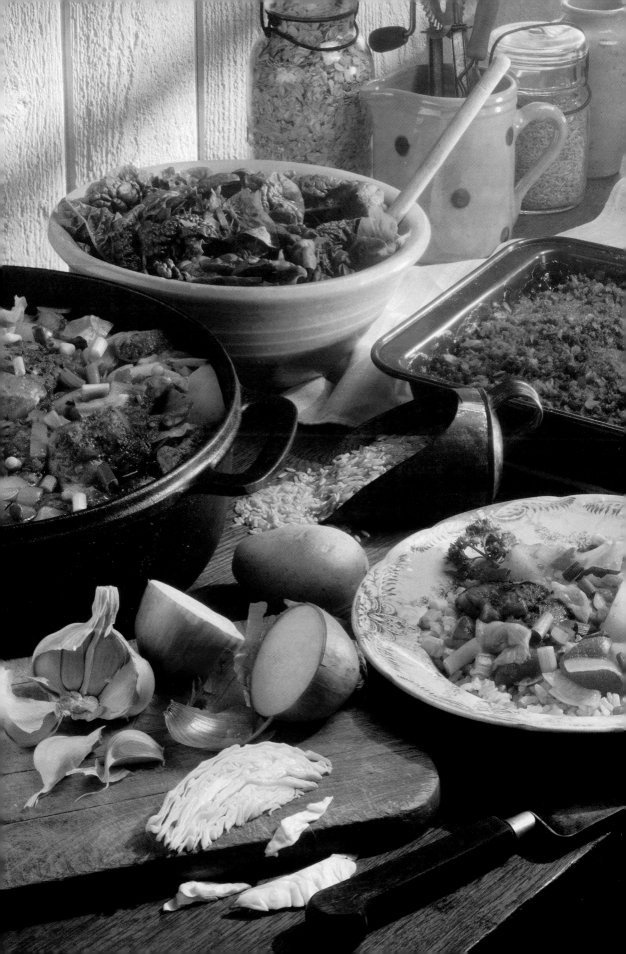

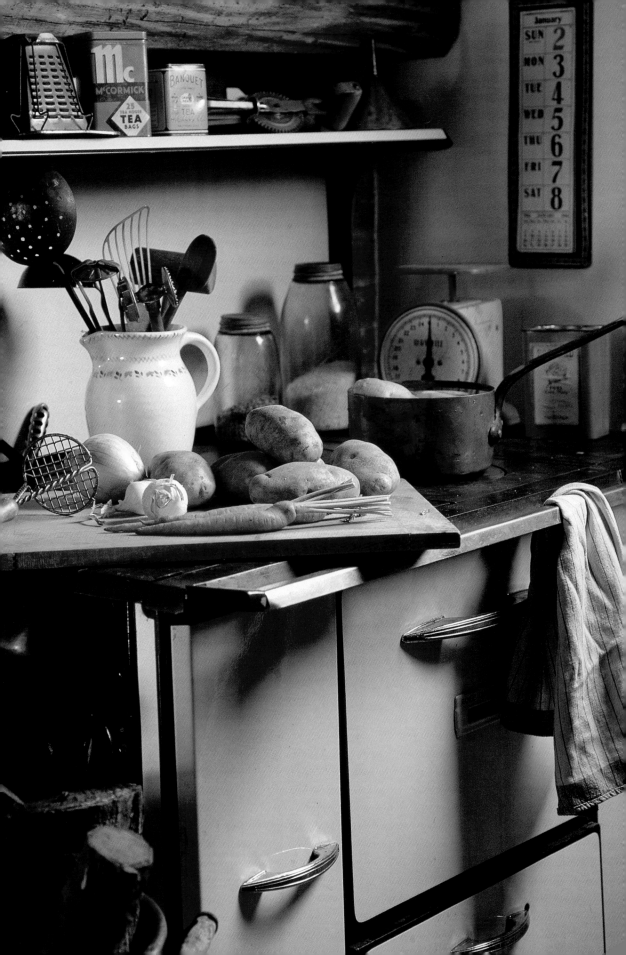

CATFISH STEW AND RICE

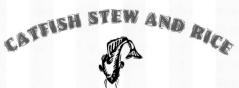

2 medium potatoes

1, 14½-oz can tomatoes,* cut up

1 cup chopped onion

1, 8-oz bottle (1 cup) clam juice or water

1 cup water

2 cloves garlic, minced

½ head cabbage, coarsely chopped

1 lb catfish fillets

1½ tbsp Hot 'N Spicy Seasoning
(see recipe below)

sliced green onion for garnish (optional)

2 cups hot cooked rice (white or brown)

Peel potatoes and cut into quarters. In a large pot combine potatoes, tomatoes and their juice, onion, clam juice, water, and garlic. Bring to boiling; reduce heat. Cook, covered, over medium-low heat for 10 minutes.

Add cabbage. Return to boiling. Reduce heat; cook, covered, over medium-low heat for 5 minutes, stirring occasionally.

Meanwhile, cut fillets into 2-inch lengths. Coat with Hot 'N Spicy Seasoning. Add fish to vegetables. Reduce heat; simmer, covered, for 5 minutes or until fish flakes easily with a fork.

Serve in soup plates, garnished with sliced green onion. Top with an ice cream scoop of hot cooked rice. Or, ladle stew over hot cooked rice in soup plates and garnish with green onion.

*To reduce sodium, try low sodium canned tomatoes

Makes 4 servings
Per serving:

calories: 355	sodium: 454 mg
total fat: 5 g	dietary fiber: 7 g
saturated fat: 1.3 g	carbohydrates: 49 g
cholesterol: 65 mg	protein: 28 g

HOT 'N SPICY SEASONING

¼ cup paprika

2 tbsp dried oregano, crushed

2 tsp chili powder

1 tsp garlic powder

1 tsp black pepper

½ tsp red (cayenne) pepper

½ tsp dry mustard

Mix together all ingredients. Store in airtight container. Makes about ⅓ cup.

MENU

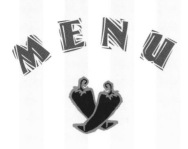

New Orleans Red Beans*

Hot Fluffy Brown Rice

Mixed Greens*

Sliced Tomatoes and Basil

Whole Grain Bread or Buns

Homemade Applesauce made with Unpeeled Apples

"Monday was laundry day in our house. Laundry day meant red beans and rice to us because we let them cook all day as we washed and starched and dried and ironed the family's clothes. We had plenty of thyme in the garden; so we used lots of that. What we didn't know then was just how healthy our Monday dinners were. Today's version, made without fat, is even healthier. It's just what the doctor ordered!"
—*Leah Chase*

*Recipe included

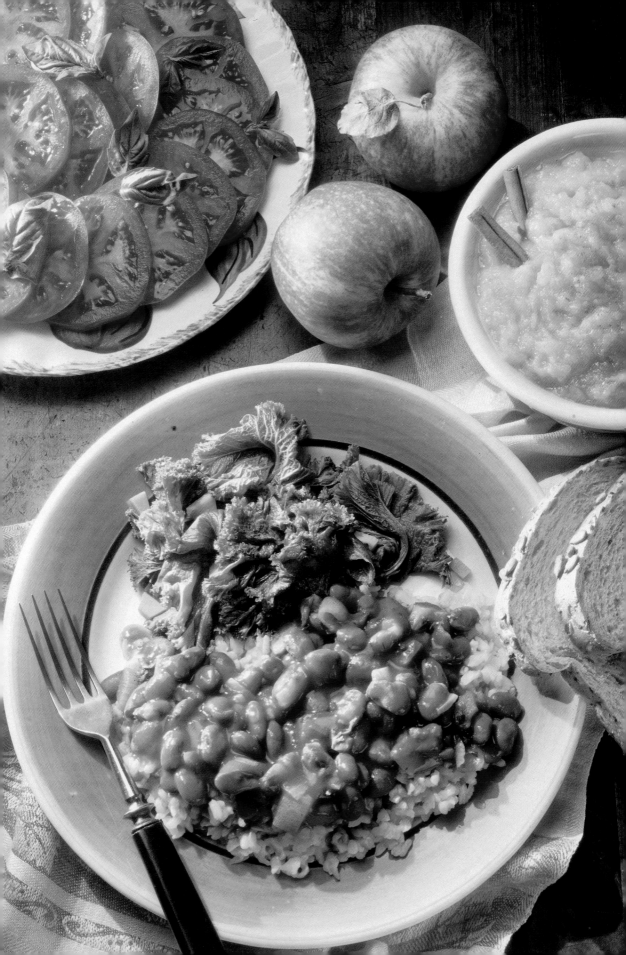

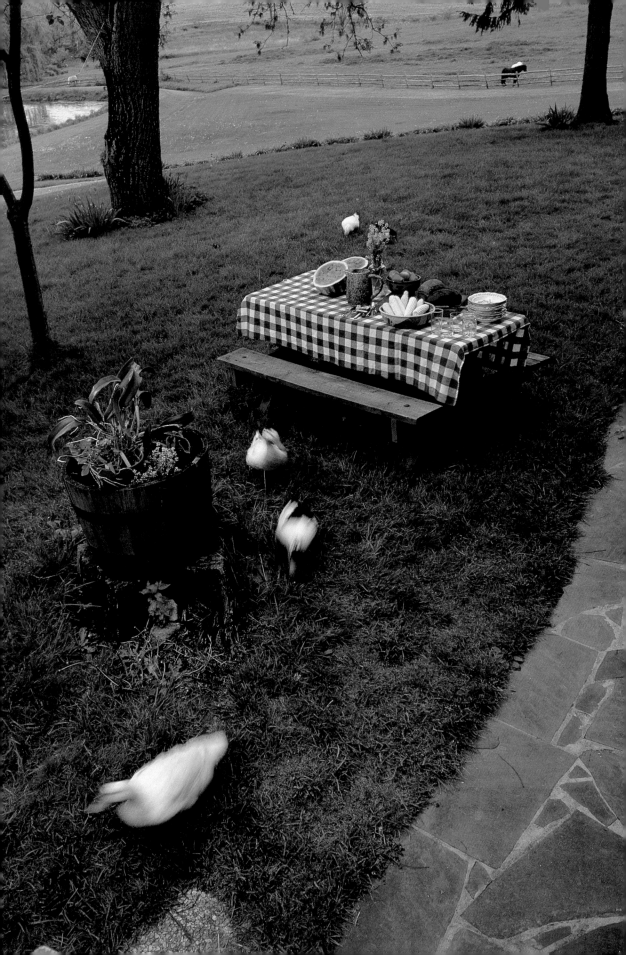

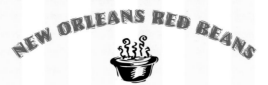

1 lb dry red beans	3 tbsp chopped garlic
2 quarts water	3 tbsp chopped parsley
1½ cups chopped onion	2 tsp dried thyme, crushed
1 cup chopped celery	1 tsp salt
4 bay leaves	1 tsp black pepper
1 cup chopped sweet green pepper	

Pick through beans to remove bad beans; rinse thoroughly. In a 5-quart pot combine beans, water, onion, celery, and bay leaves. Bring to boiling; reduce heat. Cover and cook over low heat, for about 1½ hours or until beans are tender. Stir and mash beans against side of pan.

Add green pepper, garlic, parsley, thyme, salt, and black pepper. Cook, uncovered, over low heat until creamy, about 30 minutes. Remove bay leaves. Serve over hot cooked brown rice, if desired.

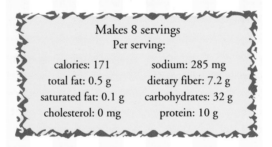

Makes 8 servings
Per serving:

calories: 171	sodium: 285 mg
total fat: 0.5 g	dietary fiber: 7.2 g
saturated fat: 0.1 g	carbohydrates: 32 g
cholesterol: 0 mg	protein: 10 g

MIXED GREENS

2 bunches mustard greens or kale	pepper to taste (optional)
2 bunches turnip greens	1 tsp salt, or to taste (optional)

Rinse greens well, removing stems. In a large pot of boiling water cook greens rapidly, covered, over medium heat for about 25 minutes or until tender. Serve with some of the pot liquor. If desired, cut greens in pan with a sharp knife and kitchen fork before serving.

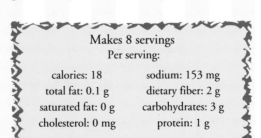

Makes 8 servings
Per serving:

calories: 18	sodium: 153 mg
total fat: 0.1 g	dietary fiber: 2 g
saturated fat: 0 g	carbohydrates: 3 g
cholesterol: 0 mg	protein: 1 g

Note: If desired, add 2 tbsp of lean cooked ham, Canadian bacon, or split turkey thighs (see page 9) to greens before serving. However, this will increase calorie, sodium, and fat content.

MENU

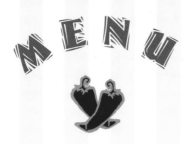

Baked Pork Chops*

Sweet Potato Custard*

Steamed Broccoli with Lemon Wedge

Cucumber with Mint and Yogurt

Winter Crisp*

*Recipe included

"Vegetables are so versatile. You'll see what I mean when you try the sweet potato custard on page 28."
—*Johnny Rivers*

"Meat is very much a part of **lean** cooking. Just remember the three C's:

• **C**hose lean cuts of meat.

• **C**ut all visible fat from meat before preparation.

• **C**ook in ways that reduce, rather than add, fat.

For example, for this recipe choose center-cut pork chops. Cut off all the fat you see, then bake, rather than fry, the breaded chops. They'll be just as juicy, just as tender as fattier, fried chops, but they'll be healthier for you and the kids."
—*Leah Chase*

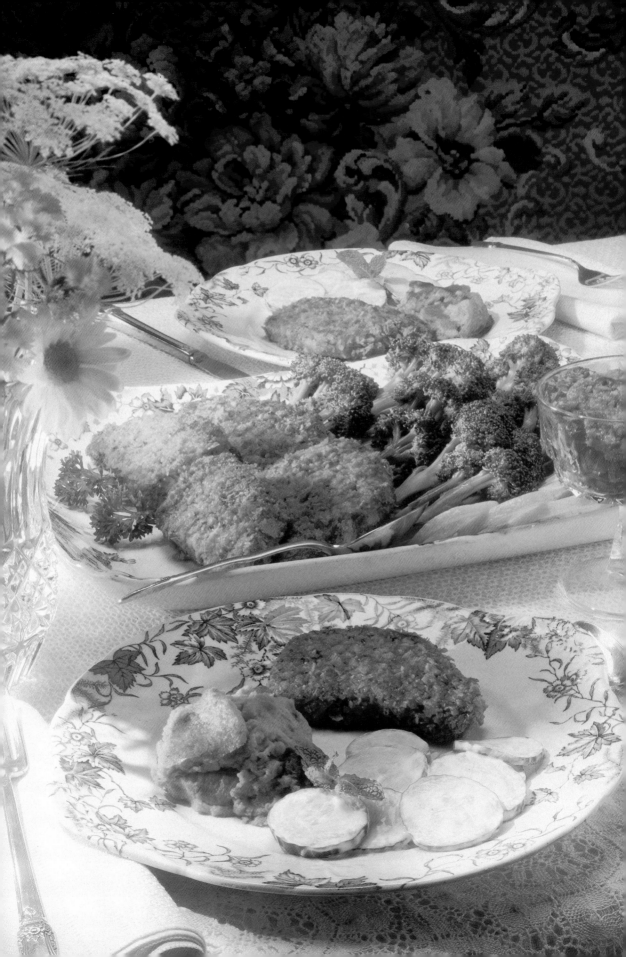

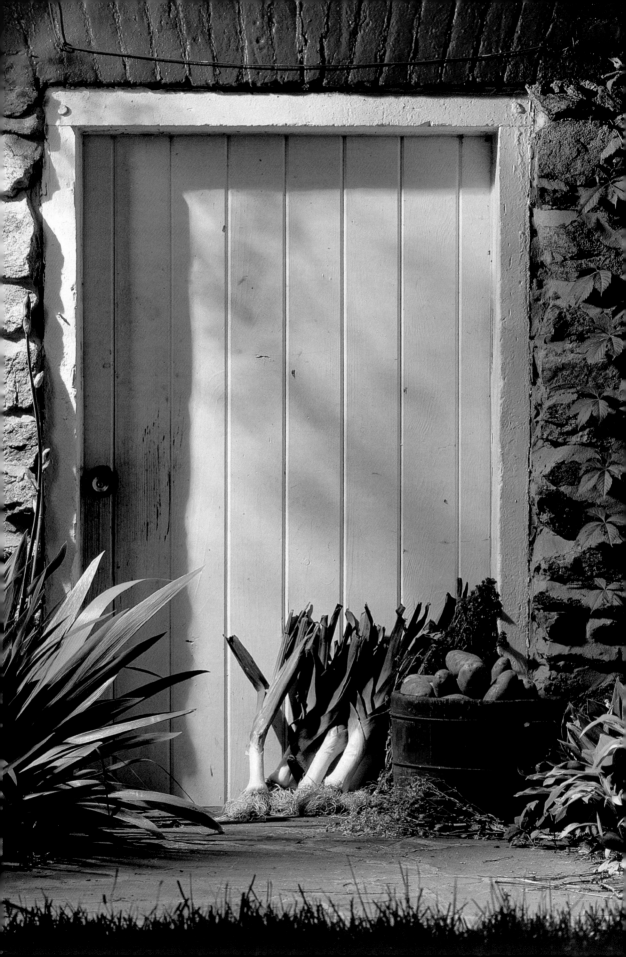

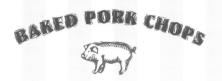

BAKED PORK CHOPS

6 lean center-cut pork chops, ½-inch thick

1 egg white

1 cup evaporated skim milk

¾ cup cornflake crumbs

¼ cup fine dry bread crumbs

2 tbsp Hot 'N Spicy Seasoning (see page 19)

½ tsp salt

Nonstick spray coating

Trim all fat from chops.

Beat egg white with evaporated skim milk. Place chops in milk mixture; let stand for 5 minutes, turning chops once.

Meanwhile, mix together cornflake crumbs, bread crumbs, Hot 'N Spicy Seasoning and salt. Remove chops from milk mixture. Coat thoroughly with crumb mixture.

Spray a 13x9-inch baking pan with nonstick spray coating. Place chops in pan; bake in 375-degree oven for 20 minutes. Turn chops; bake 15 minutes longer or till no pink remains.

Note: If desired, substitute skinless, boneless chicken, turkey pieces, or fish for pork chops and bake for 20 minutes.

Makes 6 servings
Per serving:

calories: 186	sodium: 393 mg
total fat: 4.9 g	dietary fiber: 0.2 g
saturated fat: 1.8 g	carbohydrates: 16 g
cholesterol: 31 mg	protein: 17 g

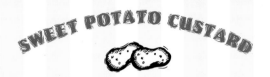

SWEET POTATO CUSTARD

1 cup mashed cooked sweet potato

½ cup mashed banana
(about 2 small)

1 cup evaporated skim milk

2 tbsp packed brown sugar

2 beaten egg yolks
(or ⅓ cup egg substitute)

½ tsp salt

¼ cup raisins

1 tbsp sugar

1 tsp ground cinnamon

Nonstick spray coating

In a medium bowl stir together sweet potato and banana. Add milk, blending well.
Add brown sugar, egg yolks, and salt, mixing thoroughly.

Spray a 1-quart casserole with nonstick spray coating.
Transfer sweet potato mixture to casserole.

Combine raisins, sugar, and cinnamon; sprinkle over top of sweet potato mixture.
Bake in a preheated 300-degree oven for 45 to 50 minutes or until
a knife inserted near center comes out clean.

Makes 6 servings
Per serving:

calories: 144	sodium: 235 mg
total fat: 2 g	dietary fiber: 1.4 g
saturated fat: 0.7 g	carbohydrates: 20 g
cholesterol: 92 mg	protein: 6 g

Note: If made with egg
substitute, the amount of
cholesterol will be lower.

WINTER CRISP

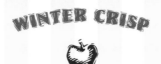

FILLING	TOPPING
½ cup sugar	⅔ cup rolled oats
3 tbsp all-purpose flour	⅓ cup packed brown sugar
1 tsp grated lemon peel	¼ cup whole wheat flour
5 cups unpeeled, sliced apples	2 tsp ground cinnamon
1 cup cranberries	3 tbsp soft margarine, melted

Filling

In a medium bowl combine sugar, flour, and lemon peel; mix well. Add apples and cranberries; stir to mix. Spoon into a 6-cup baking dish.

Topping

In a small bowl combine oats, brown sugar, flour, and cinnamon. Add melted margarine; stir to mix. Sprinkle topping over filling.

Bake in a 375-degree oven for 40 to 50 minutes or until filling is bubbly and top is brown. Serve warm or at room temperature.

SUMMER CRISP

Prepare as directed, substituting 4 cups fresh or unsweetened frozen (thawed) peaches and 2 cups fresh or unsweetened frozen (thawed) blueberries for apples and cranberries. If frozen, thaw fruit completely (do not drain).

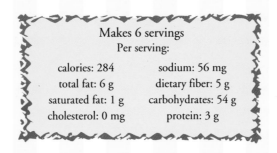

Makes 6 servings
Per serving:

calories: 284	sodium: 56 mg
total fat: 6 g	dietary fiber: 5 g
saturated fat: 1 g	carbohydrates: 54 g
cholesterol: 0 mg	protein: 3 g

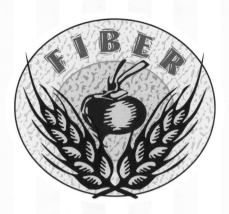

WHAT IS FIBER?

Fiber is found in the stems, seeds, leaves, and fruits of plants. Because fiber can't completely be digested, it adds bulk and therefore helps to move food waste out of the body more quickly.

WHERE'S THE FIBER?

Fiber is found only in plant foods, such as:

Whole-grain products including breads from whole wheat, rye, bran, and cornflour or cornmeal; pastas, whole-grain or bran cereals, brown rice.

Vegetables such as broccoli, brussels sprouts, cabbage, carrots, green beans and peas, lentils, dried beans and peas, sweet potato, turnip, and all forms of greens, cooked or raw.

Fruits such as apples, bananas, berries, cantaloupe, kiwi, orange, peaches, pears, watermelon and other melons, dried fruits such as raisins, dates, apricots and prunes.

Nuts and seeds (these are also high in fat).

"Growing up, my sisters and cousins and I have happy memories of Mom's meals…lots of fresh vegetables, sweet potato pie and Johnny cakes. She could do wonders with grains and beans. She used to call those things **roughage.** Now we call them **fiber.** According to National Cancer Institute studies, adult Americans don't eat much fiber—about 11 grams a day on average. But, research shows populations that eat fiber-rich foods have lower rates of colon cancer. That's why many health professionals recommend we eat twice as much fiber as we do today. A meal like this one is really on target!"

—*Johnny Rivers*

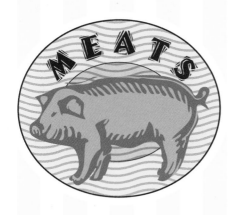

LOWER FAT CUTS OF MEAT

Beef ◆ top round ◆ eye of round ◆ round steak ◆ rump roast ◆ sirloin tip ◆ chuck arm pot roast ◆ short loin ◆ strip steak lean extra lean ground beef ◆ **Pork** ◆ tenderloin ◆ sirloin roast or chop ◆ center cut loin chops ◆ **Lamb** ◆ foreshank ◆ leg roast ◆ leg chop ◆ loin chop

MARINADE RECIPE

1 cup ketchup*

½ cup water

¼ cup vinegar

2 tbsp dry onion soup mix**

2 tbsp Worcestershire sauce (optional)

1 tbsp mustard

1 tbsp brown sugar

1 tsp chili powder

Combine marinade ingredients and heat to boiling. Cool and store in refrigerator until ready to use. Makes enough for 2 lbs of beef or pork.

To lower the salt: *Use low sodium tomato sauce instead of ketchup; and **Use one cube of low sodium broth and one teaspoon each of onion and garlic powder instead of dry onion soup mix.

"Other pork cuts to include in a healthy diet are pork loin, center-cut roast, rump or leg roasts, pork tenderloins, Canadian bacon, and shank half of ham. But remember that although Canadian Bacon and ham are low in fat, they are higher in sodium than fresh pork."

"Sometimes, less tender cuts of meat like round or rump need marinating. To add flavor and tenderize, use an oil-free marinade like the recipe on this page. Place the meat in a plastic bag set in a deep bowl; pour the marinade into the bag and tie bag closed. Marinate 1 to 2 hours at room temperature or overnight in the refrigerator. Turn bag occasionally to distribute the marinade. Do not baste with the marinade while the meat is cooking. Throw away all leftover marinade."

—*Johnny Rivers*

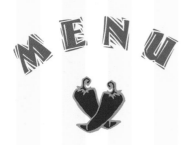

MENU

Black Skillet Beef with Greens and Red Potatoes*

Crispy Whole Wheat Rolls

Fresh Bananas and Grapes

Fig Bar Cookies

"This has everything a busy person needs. It's quick, uses only one pot, (a black cast iron skillet if you have one), it's inexpensive and tastes wonderful. I serve it in the cooking skillet, at one of the restaurants because the colors are so attractive."

"Folks who want meat can still enjoy our favorite recipes. Just plan to eat no more than two 3-ounce servings of cooked, trimmed meat (4 ounces raw) each day. I follow the 3 C's rule and I choose lower fat meats. Then I cut off all visible fat and cook it by baking, simmering, roasting, broiling, grilling, braising, microwaving, or stir frying in a nonstick skillet. All breast meat of chicken and turkey, once the skin is removed, is low in fat. —*Johnny Rivers*

*Recipe included on page 35

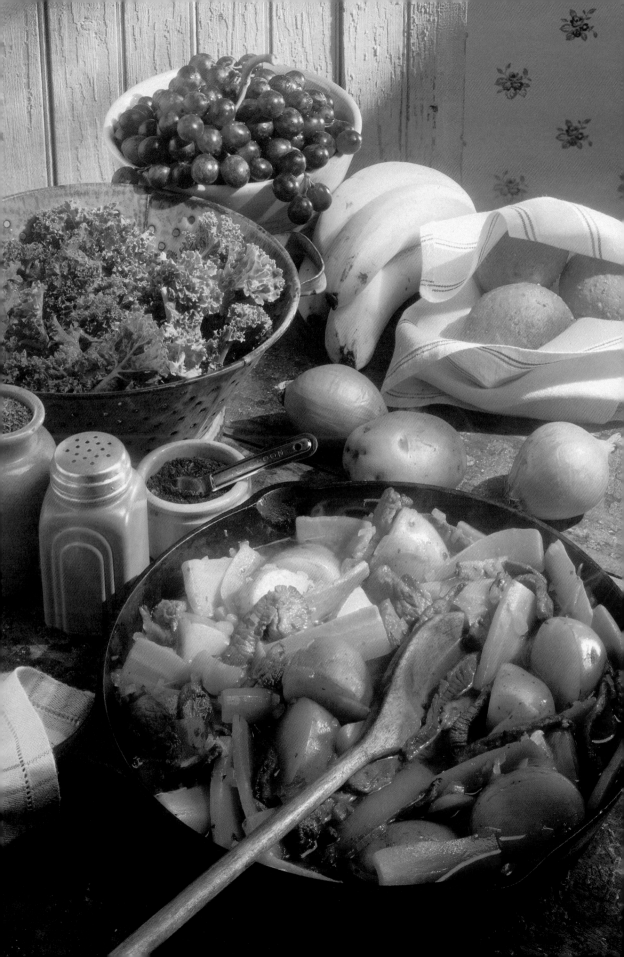

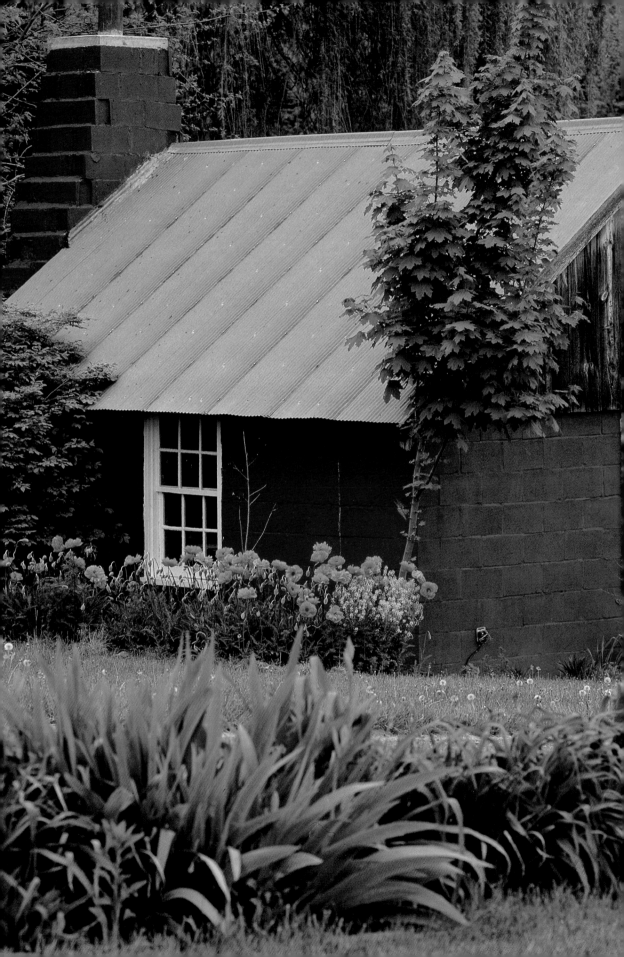

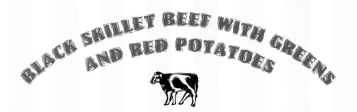

BLACK SKILLET BEEF WITH GREENS AND RED POTATOES

1 lb beef top round

1½ tbsp Hot 'N Spicy Seasoning
(see recipe on page 19)

8 red-skinned potatoes, halved

3 cups finely chopped onion

2 cups beef broth

2 large cloves garlic, minced

2 large carrots, peeled, cut into
very thin 2½-inch strips

2 bunches (½ lb each)
mustard greens, kale, or
turnip greens, stems removed,
coarsely torn

Nonstick spray coating

Partially freeze beef. Thinly slice across the grain into long strips ⅛-inch thick. Thoroughly coat strips with Hot 'N Spicy Seasoning.

Spray a large heavy skillet (cast iron is good) with nonstick spray coating. Preheat pan over high heat. Add meat; cook, stirring, for 5 minutes.

Add potatoes, onion, broth, and garlic. Cook, covered, over medium heat for 20 minutes. Stir in carrots, lay greens over top, and cook, covered, until carrots are tender, about 15 minutes. Serve in large serving bowl, with crusty bread for dunking.

Makes 6 servings
Per serving:

calories: 342	sodium: 101 mg
total fat: 4 g	dietary fiber: 10 g
saturated fat: 1.4 g	carbohydrates: 52 g
cholesterol: 45 mg	protein: 24 g

"Research suggests that in addition to fiber, other things in vegetables may help protect against cancer. Today's menu with greens, potatoes with their skins on, whole grain rolls, and fruit means that we're eating well while protecting our family's health. And that's what we care about!"— *Johnny Rivers*

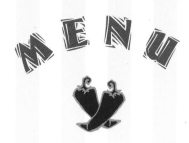

MENU

Spaghetti with Turkey* Meat Sauce

Spinach Salad with Light Garlic Dressing

Fresh Strawberries

Oatmeal Cookies

"This is my idea of comfort food. Pasta, whether hot, as in this recipe, or cold, as in the Chillin' Out Pasta Salad, (page 40) is my idea of a welcoming dish. My meat sauces have slimmed down since my early days. This turkey meat sauce is filling and rich-tasting and is a regular part of my week. Without the skin, chicken and turkey are relatively low in fat and saturated fat, which makes it my choice every time. So, remember—every time you remove the skin and fat from poultry, you're helping yourself and your family to good health."

—*Johnny Rivers*

*Recipe included on page 39.

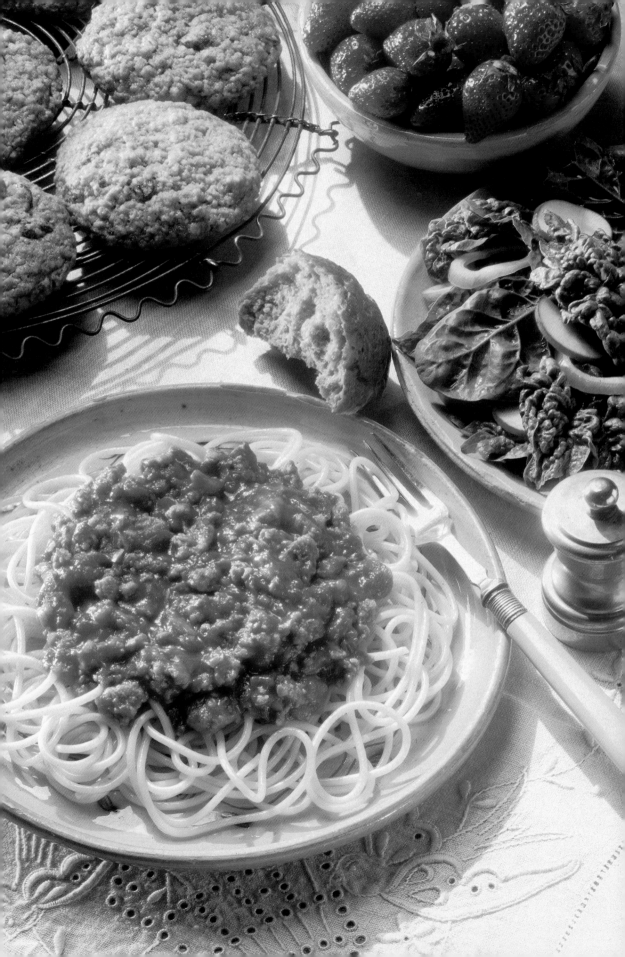

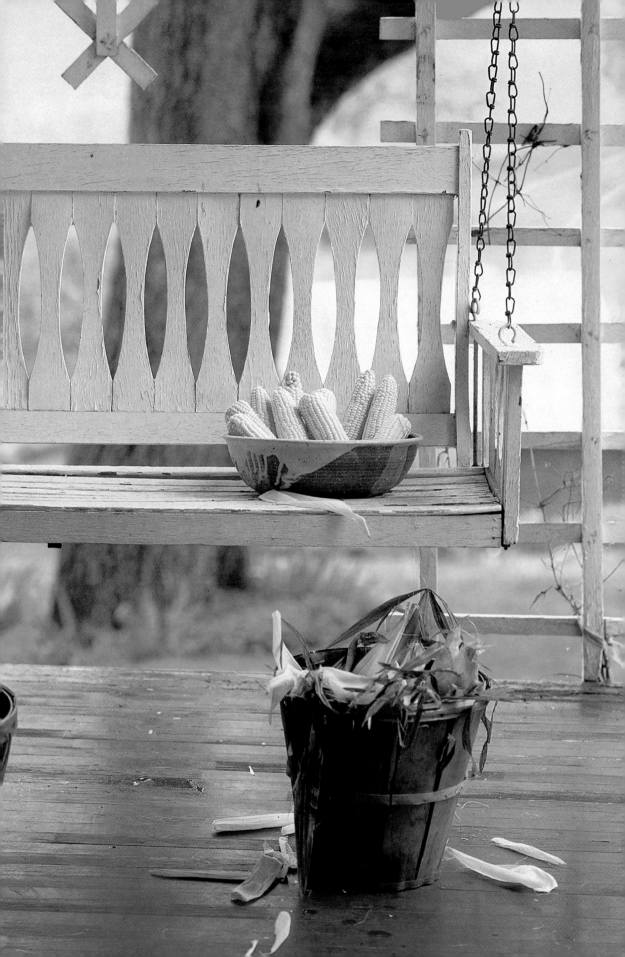

SPAGHETTI WITH TURKEY MEAT SAUCE

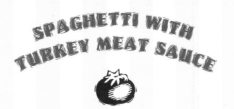

1 lb ground turkey

1, 28-oz can tomatoes, cut up

1 cup finely chopped
sweet green pepper

1 cup finely chopped onion

2 cloves garlic, minced

1 tsp dried oregano, crushed

1 tsp black pepper

1 lb spaghetti

Nonstick spray coating

Spray a large skillet with nonstick spray coating. Preheat over high heat. Add turkey; cook, stirring occasionally, for 5 minutes. Drain fat.

Stir in tomatoes with their juice, green pepper, onion, garlic, oregano, and black pepper. Bring to boiling; reduce heat. Simmer, covered, for 15 minutes, stirring occasionally.

Remove cover; simmer for 15 minutes more. (If you like a creamier sauce, give sauce a whirl in your blender or food processor.)

Meanwhile, cook spaghetti according to package directions; drain well. Serve sauce over spaghetti with your favorite crusty, whole grain bread.

Makes 6 servings
Per serving:

calories: 330	sodium: 280 mg
total fat: 5 g	dietary fiber: 2.7 g
saturated fat: 1.3 g	carbohydrates: 42 g
cholesterol: 60 mg	protein: 29 g

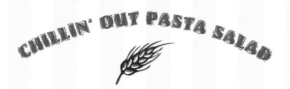

CHILLIN' OUT PASTA SALAD

8 oz (2-½ cups) medium shell pasta

1, 8-oz carton (1 cup) plain nonfat yogurt

2 tbsp spicy brown mustard

2 tbsp salt-free herb seasoning

1½ cups chopped celery

1 cup sliced green onion

1 lb cooked small shrimp

3 cups coarsely chopped tomatoes (about 3 large)

Cook pasta according to package directions. Drain; cool.

In a large bowl stir together yogurt, mustard, and herb seasoning. Add pasta, celery and green onion; mix well. Chill at least 2 hours.

Just before serving, carefully stir in shrimp and tomatoes.

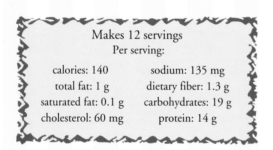

Makes 12 servings
Per serving:

calories: 140	sodium: 135 mg
total fat: 1 g	dietary fiber: 1.3 g
saturated fat: 0.1 g	carbohydrates: 19 g
cholesterol: 60 mg	protein: 14 g

"My family life was, and still is, the center of my life. Healthy food was very much a part of growing up. On the Sabbath, when I was a kid, Mom would have the table heaped with good food —vegetable loaves, broccoli casserole, cornbread made with Alabama cornmeal, and fresh fruits. So, you can see that eating lowfat is not something new. In fact, eating lowfat takes me back to my childhood. Today, our family is much larger and we only get together about once a month. We all gather at my Mom's place — often 50 to 60 people — and each one of us brings a 'covered dish.' And we play, joke, and eat well. It's important, I think, to pass on family celebrations and traditions to our kids. Now, with more knowledge about healthy eating, we know we will be protecting their health. Chillin' out pasta salad is a favorite 'covered dish' of mine." —*Johnny Rivers*

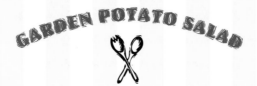

GARDEN POTATO SALAD

3 lbs potatoes (6 large)	3 tbsp lemon juice
1 cup chopped celery	2 tbsp cider vinegar
½ cup sliced green onion	½ tsp celery seed
2 tbsp chopped parsley	½ tsp dillweed
1 cup lowfat cottage cheese	½ tsp dry mustard
¾ cup skim milk	½ tsp white pepper

Scrub potatoes; boil in jackets until tender. Cool; peel. Cut into ½-inch cubes. Add celery, green onion, and parsley.

Meanwhile, in a blender, blend cottage cheese, milk, lemon juice, vinegar, celery seed, dillweed, dry mustard, and white pepper until smooth. Chill for 1 hour.

Pour chilled cottage cheese mixture over vegetables; mix well. Chill at least 30 minutes before serving.

Makes 10 servings
Per serving:

calories: 151	sodium: 118 mg
total fat: 0.5 g	dietary fiber: 3.1 g
saturated fat: 0.2 g	carbohydrates: 30 g
cholesterol: 2.3 mg	protein: 6 g

"There are 160 of us in my immediate family, and believe me, we're *family* in the best sense. Every year, we have a bang-up family party over at a friend's place in Lacombe. There's baseball, swimming, boating, fishing, water skiing, and of course, good food. Now I can share with them great tasting lowfat foods like this garden potato salad. It tastes just as good as the old fashioned kind.

P.S. If lowfat cottage cheese isn't your thing, you can substitute nonfat yogurt mixed with a bit of reduced-calorie mayonnaise for part of the dressing. For myself, I like it with the cottage cheese." —*Leah Chase*

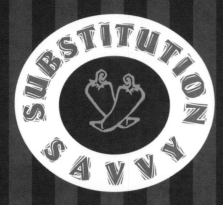

SUBSTITUTION SAVVY

You don't have to give up your favorite foods to eat a healthy diet. There are a number of ways to make the foods you love to eat lower in fat. Here are just two.

Lowfat Tip for Cooking Potatoes

Rather than home fries in butter, layer sliced potatoes (with some onion slices) in a cast iron skillet coated with no stick spray. Brush tops lightly with vegetable oil. Sprinkle with paprika and freshly cracked pepper. Roast the potatoes in the skillet in a 425 degree oven for 20 to 30 minutes or until potatoes are brown on top.

Remove the Fat

To defat homemade broths, soups and stew, prepare the food ahead and chill it. Before reheating the food, lift off the hardened fat formed at the surface. Or, if you don't have the time to chill the food, float a few ice cubes on the surface of the warm liquid to harden the fat. Then, remove the fat and discard.

When sautéing onion for flavoring stews, soups and sauces,	◈	use nonstick spray, water or stock.
When making a salad dressing,	◈	use equal parts water and vinegar and half as much oil. To make up for less intense flavor, add more mustard and herbs.
When making chocolate desserts,	◈	use 3 tablespoons of cocoa (if fat is needed to replace the fat in chocolate, add 1 tablespoon or less of vegetable oil) instead of 1 ounce of baking chocolate.
When making cakes and soft-drop cookies,	◈	use no more than 2 tablespoons of fat for each cup of flour.
When making muffins, quick breads, biscuits,	◈	use no more than 1-2 tablespoons of fat for each cup of flour.
When making muffins or quick breads,	◈	use 3 ripe, very well mashed bananas instead of ½ cup butter or oil.
When baking or cooking,	◈	use 3 egg whites and 1 yolk instead of 2 whole eggs; use 2 egg whites instead of 1 whole egg.
When making pie crust,	◈	use only ½ cup margarine for every 2 cups of flour.
When you need sour cream,	◈	blend 1 cup lowfat cottage cheese with 1 tablespoon skim milk and 2 tablespoons lemon juice, substitute plain or nonfat lowfat yogurt, or try some of the reduced fat sour cream substitutes.
When a recipe calls for butter, lard, or shortening,	◈	choose margarine with liquid vegetable oil as the first ingredient listed on the label.
To cut saturated fat,	◈	use regular soft margarine made with vegetable oil instead of butter or lard. In general, diet margarines should not be used in baking.

Here's a list of free or low-cost publications.

American Cancer Society

Eating Smart (free)

The Good Life (free)

Eat to Live (free)

To order (pending availability), call your local chapter of the American Cancer Society or call 1-800-227-2345.

American Dietetic Association

The New Cholesterol Countdown (free)

LEAN Toward Health (free)

Write: National Center for Nutrition and Dietetics, ADA, 216 W. Jackson Blvd., Suite 800, Chicago, IL 60606-6995 or call the consumer nutrition hot line 1-800-366-1655. Speak with a registered dietitian Monday-Friday 9am-4pm CST or listen to nutrition messages 24 hours daily.

American Heart Association

The American Heart Association Diet: An Eating Plan for Healthy Americans (free)

Cholesterol and Your Heart (free)

Dining Out: A Guide to Restaurant Dining (free)

How to Have Your Cake and Eat it Too (free)

Nutrition Labeling: Food Selection Hints for Fat-Controlled Meals (free)

Nutrition Nibbles (free)

Recipes for Low-Fat, Low Cholesterol Meals (free)

Write: American Heart Association, National Center, 7272 Greenville Avenue, Dallas, TX 75231. Or call 214/706-1179.

National Cancer Institute

Diet, Nutrition & Cancer Prevention: The Good News (free)

Eat More Fruits and Vegetables (free)

Easy Entertaining with Fruits and Vegetables (free)

Eat More Salads (free)

Write: Diet, Nutrition & Cancer Prevention Booklets, National Cancer Institute, Building 31, Room 10A24, Bethesda, MD 20892 or call 1-800-4-CANCER.

National Heart, Lung, and Blood Institute

So You Have High Blood Cholesterol ($1.75, stock number 017-043-00129-1)

Step by Step: Eating to Lower Your High Blood Cholesterol ($2, stock number 017-043-00130-3)

Healthy Heart Handbook for Women (NIH Publication No. 92-2720)($4.75, stock number 017-043-00122-002)

Single copies available free. For multiple copies write: Superintendent of Documents, US Government Printing Office, Washington, DC 20402. Send check, money order or use VISA or Mastercard.

Single copies of the following are available free from NHLBI Information Center, P.O. Box 30105, Bethesda, MD 20824-0105, 301-251-1222.

Facts About Blood Cholesterol (NIH Publication No. 94-2696)

Eat Right to Lower Your High Blood Cholesterol (NIH Publication No. 90-2972)

Check Your Healthy Heart I.Q. (NIH Publication No. 92-2724)

Check Your High Blood Pressure Prevention I.Q. (NIH Publication No. 94-3671)

Check Your Weight and Heart Disease I.Q. (NIH Publication No. 90-3034)

Exercise and Your Heart–A Guide to Physical Activity (NIH Publication No. 93-1677)

Facts About How to Prevent High Blood Pressure (NIH Publication No. 94-3281)

Eat Right to Help Lower Your High Blood Pressure (NIH Publication No. 92-3289)

High Blood Pressure: Treat It for Life (NIH Publication No. 94-3312)

U.S. Department of Agriculture/U.S. Department of Health and Human Services

Nutrition and Your Health: Dietary Guidelines for Americans (HG-232, single copies 50 cents).

Write: Consumer Information Center, Department 314-A, Pueblo, CO 81009.

U.S. Department of Agriculture

Dietary Guidelines and Your Diet (HG-253-1 through 8, $6.50 for eight bulletins, stock number 001-000-04598-9).

Preparing Foods and Planning Menus Using the Dietary Guidelines ($2.50, stock number 001-000-045427-0)

Making Bag Lunches, Snacks and Desserts Using the Dietary Guidelines ($2.50, stock number 001-000-04528-8)

Shopping for Food and Making Meals in Minutes Using the Dietary Guidelines ($3.00, stock number 001-000-04529-6)

Eating Better When Eating Out Using the Dietary Guidelines ($1.50, stock number 001-000-04530-0)

Write: Superintendent of Documents, US Government Printing Office, Washington, DC 20402. Make check or money order payable to the Superintendent of Documents or call 202/783-3238. Orders may be charged to VISA or Mastercard.